T0162628

STRESS RELEASE
in 5 Minutes a Day
★★★ *through* ★★★
AMERICAN
WISDOM

★★★

JOHN KERECZ

ⅭiUniverse®

STRESS RELEASE IN 5 MINUTES A DAY
THROUGH AMERICAN WISDOM

iUniverse books may be ordered through booksellers or by contacting:

iUniverse
1663 Liberty Drive
Bloomington, IN 47403
www.iuniverse.com
1-800-Authors (1-800-288-4677)

ISBN: 978-1-4917-9739-6 (sc)
ISBN: 978-1-4917-9740-2 (e)

Print information available on the last page.

iUniverse rev. date: 05/17/2016

"One's destination is never a place, but a new way of seeing things."

--Henry Miller

CONTENTS

A special thanks goes out to Christine Robbins for not only editing this book but for being my friend.

I'd like to dedicate this book to my love Janice Marie who has shown me that there is a lot more to life than I thought.

FOREWORD

The need for contemplative thought and critical thinking is greater than ever. The constant barrage of life's demands and cultural information has left us with very little time to reflect on what it all may mean to us and to our world. The practice of meditation has more to offer us than ever, just when we have the least time and awareness to devote to it. That is the beauty and simplicity of this book. By selecting and arranging just one quote per day, the author has distilled the wisdom of 240 years into easily digestible bites. By taking the time each day to contemplate the quotes within this book, we can begin to understand more about ourselves and other people. Whether you've practiced meditation for years or the concept is new to you, this book provides a template to map your journey or launch your exploration. How does a witticism from Mark Twain apply to internet dating? What advice can Benjamin Franklin offer to help us deal with road rage? The answers are within you. Take the time, just five minutes each day, to know yourself and these prominent Americans better.

Chris Robbins

INTRODUCTION

I'm going to make this introduction shorter than those of my other books. This is the third in a planned trilogy of books all dealing with stress release. My first was filled with Zen principles. My second with Biblical verse. And now this one, compiling American philosophy and wisdom. The sayings I've included are from our founding fathers, past presidents, iconic entertainers, and writers. All of my books promote Ascentology, the idea that you work to "ascend" at your own pace to better yourself. The focus here is that by taking just five minutes a day to think about a particular quote and how it might apply to your life, the stress of your life will be reduced. You may consider that contemplation or meditation. In my other books I went over some basic ways to meditate, the only thing I'd like to add here is that meditation can coincide with a body in motion. You may choose to sit by yourself and think about the quote, or read it in the morning and think about it throughout the day, while at work or play, or while driving on your commute. The page underneath each quote has space for you to write your thoughts. You may choose to write your thoughts as soon as you read each saying, or you can write your thoughts the next day before you turn the page. You can add notes throughout the day as your contemplation deepens and changes. Focusing on something and recording your thoughts and feelings is an easy concept of self-help. These quotes are to help you on your journey -- what you get out of it is up to you. I've included 365 quotes, one for each day of the year.

Since my last publication, my life itself has changed. I've traveled more and learned to enjoy my life more. Contemplation and meditation are things that I take with me and my approach to them changes as I do. Your meditation doesn't have to be the traditional kind of meditation, but instead whatever makes you feel better, however you can release your stress and relax in this day and age. I've noticed a big change in our society since the publication of my last book, people are busier than ever and crave instant results; quicker gratification in less time. That is why I added the "five minutes a day" concept and title to this book. Five minutes is all the time you really need to find yourself and learn how to center yourself and relax throughout the day and find peace. I hope these sayings give you something to think about and help you with your life and hopefully encourage you to pick up my other books. I wish you luck on your journey and I hope these daily reflections help you to better your life!

John J. Kerecz

The jaws of power are always open to devour, and her arm is always stretched out, if possible, to destroy the freedom of thinking, speaking, and writing.

--John Adams

If ever time should come, when vain and aspiring men shall possess the highest seats in Government, our country will stand in need of its experienced patriots to prevent its ruin.

--Samuel Adams

You know that being an American is more than a matter of where your parents came from. It is a belief that all men are created free and equal and that everyone deserves an even break.

--*Harry S Truman*

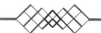

Those who expect to reap the blessings of freedom, must, like men, undergo the fatigue of supporting it.

--James Madison

"Classic." A book which people praise and don't read.

--Mark Twain

If everyone is thinking alike, then somebody isn't thinking.

--George S. Patton

The whole world is bound together as never before; the bonds are sometimes those of hatred rather than love, but they are bonds nevertheless. Frowning or hopeful, every man of leadership in any line of thought or effort must now look beyond the limits of his own country.

--Theodore Roosevelt

Trust, but verify.

--Ronald Reagan

You don't lead by hitting people over the head - that's assault, not leadership.

--Dwight D. Eisenhower

If I am killed, I can die but once; but to live in constant dread of it, is to die over and over again.

--Abraham Lincoln

The test of our progress is not whether we add more to the abundance of those who have much; it is whether we provide enough for those who have too little.

--Franklin D. Roosevelt

A bone to the dog is not charity. Charity is the bone shared with the dog, when you are just as hungry as the dog.

--Jack London

You can't get away from yourself by moving from one place to another.

--Ernest Hemingway

If there is one thing which I would banish from the earth it is fear.

--Henry Ford

...'tis easier to keep holidays than commandments.

--Benjamin Franklin

The man who reads nothing at all is better educated than the man who reads nothing but newspapers.

--Thomas Jefferson

A bureaucrat is a Democrat who holds some office that a Republican wants.

--Harry S Truman

Great thoughts speak only to the thoughtful mind, but great actions speak to all mankind.

--*Theodore Roosevelt*

If we were sensible we would seek death--the same blissful blank which we enjoyed before we existed.

--H. P. Lovecraft

The only thing worse than being blind is having sight but no vision.

--Hellen Keller

Voting is easy and marginally useful, but it is a poor substitute for democracy, which requires direct action by concerned citizens.

--Howard Zinn

Towering genius disdains a beaten path. It seeks regions hitherto unexplored.

--Abraham Lincoln

You can't build a reputation on what you are going to do.

--Henry Ford

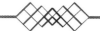

If you could kick the person in the pants responsible for most of your trouble, you wouldn't sit for a month.

--*Theodore Roosevelt*

To the scientist there is the joy in pursuing truth which nearly counteracts the depressing revelations of truth.

--H. P. Lovecraft

A little integrity is better than any career.

--*Ralph Waldo Emerson*

I have been driven many times upon my knees by the overwhelming conviction that I had nowhere else to go. My own wisdom, and that of all about me, seemed insufficient for the day.

--*Abraham Lincoln*

In order to make a man or a boy covet a thing, it is only necessary to make the thing difficult to obtain.

--*Mark Twain*

Nothing can now be believed which is seen in a newspaper. Truth itself becomes suspicious by being put into that polluted vehicle.

--Thomas Jefferson

The ultimate measure of a man is not where he stands in moments of comfort and convenience, but where he stands at times of challenge and controversy.

--Martin Luther King, Jr.

You can observe a lot by watching.

--Yogi Berra

A business that makes nothing but money is a poor business.

--Henry Ford

Hold on, my friends, to the Constitution and to the Republic for which it stands. Miracles do not cluster, and what has happened once in 6000 years, may not happen again.

--*Theodore Roosevelt*

It was my fortune, or misfortune, to be called to the office of Chief Executive without any previous political training.

--Ulysses S. Grant

People like you to be something, preferably what they are.

--John Steinbeck

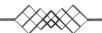

To be able to forget means sanity.

--Jack London

Necessity never made a good bargain.

--Benjamin Franklin

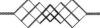

Some men can live up to their loftiest ideals without ever going higher than a basement.

--*Theodore Roosevelt*

The very ink with which all history is written is merely fluid prejudice.

--Mark Twain

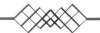

Without morals a republic cannot subsist any length of time

--Samuel Adams

A conservative is a man with two perfectly good legs who, however, has never learned to walk forward.

--Franklin D. Roosevelt

Pull the string, and it will follow wherever you wish. Push it, and it will go nowhere at all.

--Dwight D. Eisenhower

Wise men have interpreted dreams, and the gods have laughed.

--H. P. Lovecraft

It's a hard thing to leave any deeply routine life, even if you hate it.

--*John Steinbeck*

In skating over thin ice, our safety is in our speed.

--Ralph Waldo Emerson

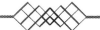

Much of the usefulness of any career must lie in the impress that it makes upon, and the lessons that it teaches to, the generations that come after.

--Theodore Roosevelt

Thinking is the hardest work there is, which is probably the reason so few engage in it.

--Henry Ford

In those wretched countries where a man cannot call his tongue his own, he can scarce call anything his own. Whoever would overthrow the liberty of a nation must begin by subduing the freeness of speech.

--Benjamin Franklin

The struggle for today is not altogether for today -- it is for a vast future also.

--Abraham Lincoln

A little rebellion now and then is a good thing and as necessary in the political world as storms in the physical.

--*Thomas Jefferson*

In the End, we will remember not the words of our enemies, but the silence of our friends.

--*Martin Luther King, Jr.*

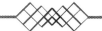

Who ever hears of fat men heading a riot, or herding together in turbulent mobs? — No — no, 'tis your lean, hungry men who are continually worrying society, and setting the whole community by the ears.

--*Washington Irving*

A man is never more truthful than when he acknowledges himself a liar.

--Mark Twain

The thing worse than rebellion is the thing that causes rebellion.

--Frederick Douglass

Research is creating new knowledge.

--Neil Armstrong

Injustice anywhere is a threat to justice everywhere.

--Martin Luther King, Jr.

Far better it is to dare mighty things, to win glorious triumphs, even though checkered by failure, than to rank with those poor spirits who neither enjoy much nor suffer much, because they live in that grey twilight that knows neither victory nor defeat.

--Theodore Roosevelt

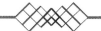

The difference between the almost right word and the right word is really a large matter—'tis the difference between the lightning-bug and the lightning.

--Mark Twain

We must use time as a tool, not as a couch.

--John F. Kennedy

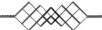

Age wrinkles the body. Quitting wrinkles the soul.

--Douglas MacArthur

We believe that if men have the talent to invent new machines that put men out of work, they have the talent to put those men back to work.

--John F. Kennedy

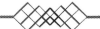

Everybody is ignorant, only on different subjects.

--Will Rogers

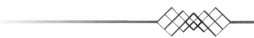

The worst loneliness is to not be comfortable with yourself.

--Mark Twain

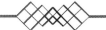

A man who has never gone to school may steal from a freight car; but if he has a university education, he may steal the whole railroad.

--Theodore Roosevelt

The religion of one age is the literary entertainment of the next.

--Ralph Waldo Emerson

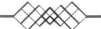

Nothing that grieves us can be called little: by the eternal laws of proportion a child's loss of a doll and a king's loss of a crown are events of the same size.

--*Mark Twain*

The problem in defense is how far you can go without destroying from within what you are trying to defend from without.

--Dwight D. Eisenhower

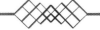

Philanthropy is commendable, but it must not cause the philanthropist to overlook the circumstances of economic injustice which make philanthropy necessary.

--Martin Luther King, Jr.

It is always possible to do a thing better the second time.

--Henry Ford

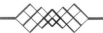

Creativity is just connecting things. When you ask creative people how they did something, they feel a little guilty because they didn't really do it, they just saw something. It seemed obvious to them after a while. That's because they were able to connect experiences they've had and synthesize new things.

--*Steve Jobs*

A man ought to be able to live on a scale commensurate with the service that he renders.

--Henry Ford

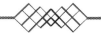

Whenever you find yourself on the side of the majority, it is time to pause and reflect.

--*Mark Twain*

In any moment of decision, the best thing you can do is the right thing, the next best thing is the wrong thing, and the worst thing you can do is nothing.

--Theodore Roosevelt

America will never be destroyed from the outside. If we falter and lose our freedoms, it will be because we destroyed ourselves.

--Thomas Jefferson

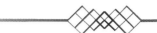

Intelligent men are cruel. Stupid men are monstrously cruel.

--Jack London

The greatest human achievements have never been for profit.

--H. P. Lovecraft

Nothing astonishes men so much as common sense and plain dealing.

--Ralph Waldo Emerson

Don't think you are going to conceal thoughts by concealing evidence that they ever existed.

--Dwight D. Eisenhower

When you're curious, you find lots of interesting things to do.

--Walt Disney

The bitterest tragic element in life to be derived from an intellectual source is the belief in a brute Fate or Destiny.

--Ralph Waldo Emerson

Silence is not always a sign of wisdom, but babbling is ever a mark of folly.

--Benjamin Franklin

Nobody cares how much you know, until they know how much you care.

--Theodore Roosevelt

It is the duty of the patriot to protect his country from its government.

--*Thomas Paine*

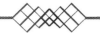

There never was a time when, in my opinion, some way could not be found to prevent the drawing of the sword.

--Ulysses S. Grant

Society is like a lawn, where every roughness is smoothed, every bramble eradicated, and where the eye is delighted by the smiling verdure of a velvet surface. He, however, who would study nature in its wildness and variety must plunge into the forest, must explore the glen, must stem the torrent, and dare the precipice.

--*Washington Irving*

All the world is full of suffering. It is also full of overcoming.

--Hellen Keller

The only saving grace of the present is that it's too damned stupid to question the past very closely.

--H. P. Lovecraft

As we must account for every idle word, so we must for every idle silence.

--Benjamin Franklin

Whenever people are well-informed they can be trusted with their own government.

--Thomas Jefferson

A question is a trap, and an answer your foot in it.

--John Steinbeck

If we desire to avoid insult, we must be able to repel it; if we desire to secure peace, one of the most powerful instruments of our rising prosperity, it must be known, that we are at all times ready for war.

--*George Washington*

We may have all come on different ships, but we're in the same boat now.

--Martin Luther King, Jr.

A people that values its privileges above its principles soon loses both.

--*Dwight D. Eisenhower*

When you play, play hard; when you work, don't play at all.

--Theodore Roosevelt

A nation that continues year after year to spend more money on military defense than on programs of social uplift is approaching spiritual doom.

--Martin Luther King, Jr.

Wealth is nothing more or less than a tool to do things with. It is like the fuel that runs the furnace or the belt that runs the wheel -- only a means to an end.

--*Henry Ford*

Self-approval is acquired mainly from the approval of other people.

--*Mark Twain*

It isn't enough to talk about peace. One must believe in it. And it isn't enough to believe in it. One must work at it.

--*Eleanor Roosevelt*

All the president is, is a glorified public relations man who spends his time flattering, kissing, and kicking people to get them to do what they are supposed to do anyway.

--Harry S Truman

Life is not the unique property of Earth. Nor is life in the shape of human beings. Life takes many forms on other planets and far stars, forms that would seem bizarre to humans, as human life is bizarre to other life-forms.

--*H. P. Lovecraft*

Self-trust is the first secret of success.

--Ralph Waldo Emerson

The only motive that can keep politics pure is the motive of doing good for one's country and its people.

--*Henry Ford*

We must especially beware of that small group of selfish men who would clip the wings of the American Eagle in order to feather their own nests.

--*Franklin D. Roosevelt*

A pessimist is one who makes difficulties of his opportunities and an optimist is one who makes opportunities of his difficulties.

--Harry S Truman

'Tis easier to suppress the first Desire, than to satisfy all that follow it.

--Benjamin Franklin

He who makes an assertion without knowing whether it is true or false, is guilty of falsehood; and the accidental truth of the assertion, does not justify or excuse him.

--Abraham Lincoln

It takes great courage to back truth unacceptable to our times.
There's a punishment for it, and it's usually crucifixion.

--John Steinbeck

Remember always that you not only have the right to be an individual, you have an obligation to be one.

--*Eleanor Roosevelt*

These libraries should be open to all -- except the censor.

--John F. Kennedy

Stay hungry, stay foolish.

--Steve Jobs

A vote is like a rifle; its usefulness depends upon the character of the user.

--Theodore Roosevelt

It cannot be emphasized too strongly or too often that this great nation was founded, not by religionists, but by Christians; not on religions, but on the Gospel of Jesus Christ. For this very reason peoples of other faiths have been afforded asylum, prosperity, and freedom of worship here.

--*Patrick Henry*

What good is the warmth of summer, without the cold of winter
to give it sweetness.

--*John Steinbeck*

Accept whatever situation you cannot improve.

--Tennessee Williams

If destruction be our lot, we must ourselves be its author and finisher. As a nation of freemen, we must live through all time, or die by suicide.

--Abraham Lincoln

When you have worn out your shoes, the strength of the shoe leather has passed into the fiber of your body. I measure your health by the number of shoes and hats and clothes you have worn out.

--Ralph Waldo Emerson

All my life, whenever it comes time to make a decision, I make it and forget about it.

--Harry S Truman

Government always finds a need for whatever money it gets.

--Ronald Reagan

Unlike presidential administrations, problems rarely have terminal dates.

--Dwight D. Eisenhower

The god of Victory is said to be one-handed, but Peace gives victory to both sides.

--Ralph Waldo Emerson

Its name is Public Opinion. It is held in reverence. It settles everything. Some think it is the voice of God.

--Mark Twain

When you have an efficient government, you have a dictatorship.

--Harry S Truman

All progress is precarious, and the solution of one problem brings us face to face with another problem.

--Martin Luther King, Jr.

Laws too gentle are seldom obeyed; too severe, seldom executed.

--Benjamin Franklin

To sin by silence when they should protest makes cowards of men.

--Abraham Lincoln

What we have once enjoyed we can never lose. All that we love deeply becomes a part of us.

--Hellen Keller

The secret of success is making your vocation your vacation.

--Mark Twain

But a constitution of government once changed from freedom, can never be restored. Liberty, once lost, is lost forever.

--John Adams

All wars are follies, very expensive, and very mischievous ones.

--*Benjamin Franklin*

The giving of love is an education in itself.

--*Eleanor Roosevelt*

When you can't make them see the light, make them feel the heat.

--Ronald Reagan

Almost always, the creative dedicated minority has made the world better.

--Martin Luther King, Jr.

It seems to me that if you or I must choose between two courses of thought or action, we should remember our dying and try so to live that our death brings no pleasure on the world.

--John Steinbeck

The day will come when the mystical generation of Jesus, by the Supreme Being as His Father, in the womb of a virgin, will be classed with the fable of the generation of Minerva, in the brain of Jupiter.

--Thomas Jefferson

When you are right you cannot be too radical; when you are wrong, you cannot be too conservative.

--Martin Luther King, Jr.

Almost nobody dances sober, unless they happen to be insane.

--H. P. Lovecraft

Intoxicated with unbroken success, we have become too self-sufficient to feel the necessity of redeeming and preserving grace, too proud to pray to the God that made us.

--Abraham Lincoln

No sane man can be happy, for to him life is real, and he sees what a fearful thing it is. Only the mad can be happy, and not many of those. The few that imagine themselves kings or gods are happy, the rest are no happier than the sane.

--*Mark Twain*

There is a certain relief in change, even though it be from bad to worse; as I have found in travelling in a stage-coach, that it is often a comfort to shift one's position and be bruised in a new place.

--Washington Irving

When you are asked if you can do a job, tell 'em, 'Certainly I can!' Then get busy and find out how to do it.

--Theodore Roosevelt

All war is a symptom of man's failure as a thinking animal.

--*John Steinbeck*

Every man alone is sincere. At the entrance of a second person, hypocrisy begins.

--Ralph Waldo Emerson

It is by the goodness of God that in our country we have those three unspeakably precious things: freedom of speech, freedom of conscience, and the prudence never to practice either.

--*Mark Twain*

Don't judge of man's wealth or piety, by their Sunday appearances.

--*Benjamin Franklin*

When the weather is good for crops it is also good for weeds.

--Theodore Roosevelt

Americans [have] the right and advantage of being armed, unlike the citizens of other countries whose governments are afraid to trust their people with arms.

--James Madison

Freedom is never voluntarily given by the oppressor; it must be demanded by the oppressed.

--Martin Luther King, Jr.

I used to say that Politics is the second oldest profession [prostitution being the oldest], but I have come to realize that it bears a gross similarity to the first.

--*William Penn*

The Constitution is not an instrument for the government to restrain the people, it is an instrument for the people to restrain the government — lest it come to dominate our lives and interests.

--*Patrick Henry*

When we remember that we are all mad, the mysteries disappear and life stands explained.

--*Mark Twain*

An idealist is a person who helps other people to be prosperous.

--Henry Ford

Drink does not drown care, but waters it, and makes it grow faster.

--Benjamin Franklin

It's not right to respond to terrorism by terrorizing other people.

--Howard Zinn

There is no security on this earth; there is only opportunity.

--Douglas MacArthur

Never confuse movement with action.

--Ernest Hemingway

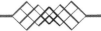

There are as many opinions as there are experts.

--Franklin D. Roosevelt

When Nature has work to be done, she creates a genius to do it.

--*Ralph Waldo Emerson*

Any humane and reasonable person must conclude that if the ends, however desirable, are uncertain and the means are horrible and certain, these means must not be employed.

--Howard Zinn

Don't let yesterday use up too much of today.

--Will Rogers

Man is an imitative animal. This quality is the germ of all education in him. From his cradle to his grave he is learning to do what he sees others do.

--*Thomas Jefferson*

The money powers prey upon the nation in times of peace and conspire against it in times of adversity. The banking powers are more despotic than a monarchy, more insolent than autocracy, more selfish than bureaucracy. They denounce as public enemies all who question their methods or throw light upon their crimes.

--Abraham Lincoln

Whatever America hopes to bring to pass in the world must first come to pass in the heart of America.

--*Dwight D. Eisenhower*

Any man's life, told truly, is a novel.

--Ernest Hemingway

I never gave anybody hell! I just told the truth and they thought it was hell.

--Harry S Truman

Nearly all men can stand adversity, but if you want to test a man's character, give him power.

--Abraham Lincoln

People who have no mind can easily be steadfast and firm...

--Mark Twain

The time is always right to do what is right.

--Martin Luther King, Jr.

When a nation issues ultimatums, it leaves no room for compromise and ensures that war will continue.

--Howard Zinn

Any people that would give up liberty for a little temporary safety deserves neither liberty nor safety.

--*Benjamin Franklin*

Do what you can, with what you have, where you are.

--Theodore Roosevelt

In great contests each party claims to act in accordance with the will of God. Both may be, and one must be, wrong. God cannot be for and against the same thing at the same time.

--*Abraham Lincoln*

Our fathers were brought hither by their high veneration for the Christian religion. They journeyed by its light, and labored in its hope. They sought to incorporate its principles with the elements of their society, and to diffuse its influence through all their institutions, civil, political, or literary.

--*Daniel Webster*

Travel is fatal to prejudice, bigotry, and narrow-mindedness, and many of our people need it sorely on these accounts.

--Mark Twain

When a man says he does not want to speak of something he usually means he can think of nothing else.

--John Steinbeck

As human beings, our only sensible scale of values is one based on lessening the agony of existence.

--H. P. Lovecraft

Courage - a perfect sensibility of the measure of danger, and a
mental willingness to endure it.

--*William Tecumseh Sherman*

If men are so wicked as we now see them with religion what would they be if without it?

--*Benjamin Franklin*

The proper function of man is to live, not to exist. I shall not waste my days in trying to prolong them. I shall use my time.

--*Jack London*

When a man assumes a public trust, he should consider himself as public property.

--Thomas Jefferson

Avarice, ambition, revenge, or gallantry, would break the strongest cords of our Constitution as a whale goes through a net.

--*John Adams*

Bad men cannot make good citizens.

--Patrick Henry

Happiness is not a goal; it is a by-product.

--Eleanor Roosevelt

If you want to succeed you should strike out on new paths,
rather than travel the worn paths of accepted success.

--John D. Rockefeller

Nonviolence is a powerful and just weapon, which cuts without wounding and ennobles the man who wields it. It is a sword that heals.

--*Martin Luther King, Jr.*

The term "just war" contains an internal contradiction. War is inherently unjust, and the great challenge of our time is how to deal with evil, tyranny, and oppression without killing huge numbers of people.

--Howard Zinn

What we call evil, it seems to me, is simply ignorance bumping its head in the dark.

--Henry Ford

Before a standing army can rule, the people must be disarmed; as they are in almost every kingdom in Europe. The supreme power in America cannot enforce unjust laws by the sword; because the whole body of the people are armed, and constitute a force superior to any band of regular troops that can be, on any pretence [sic], raised in the United States.

--Noah Webster

It may be true that he travels farthest who travels alone, but the goal thus reached is not worth reaching.

--Theodore Roosevelt

I have always thought that all men should be free; but if any should be slaves, it should first be those who desire it for themselves, and secondly those who desire it for others.

--Abraham Lincoln

My model for business is The Beatles: They were four guys that kept each others' negative tendencies in check; they balanced each other. And the total was greater than the sum of the parts.

--*Steve Jobs*

Since all motives at bottom are selfish and ignoble, we may judge acts and qualities only by their effects.

--H. P. Lovecraft

The only things worth learning are the things you learn after you know it all.

--*Harry S Truman*

We sink to rise.

--Ralph Waldo Emerson

Being against evil doesn't make you good.

--Ernest Hemingway

Capitalism does not permit an even flow of economic resources. With this system, a small privileged few are rich beyond conscience, and almost all others are doomed to be poor at some level.

--Martin Luther King, Jr.

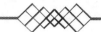

Every difference of opinion is not a difference of principle.

--Thomas Jefferson

If the world was perfect, it wouldn't be.

--Yogi Berra

It's kind of fun to do the impossible.

--Walt Disney

Remember, democracy never lasts long. It soon wastes, exhausts, and murders itself.

--John Adams

The future belongs to those who believe in the beauty of their dreams.

--Eleanor Roosevelt

We must learn to live together as brothers or perish together as fools.

--Martin Luther King, Jr.

Caged birds accept each other but flight is what they long for.

--Tennessee Williams

Democracy is two wolves and a lamb voting on what to have for lunch. Liberty is a well-armed lamb contesting the vote!

--Benjamin Franklin

Grief can take care of itself; but to get the full value of a joy you must have someone to divide it with.

--Mark Twain

If you can't convince them, confuse them.

--Harry S Truman

It would be absurd if we did not understand both angels and
devils, since we invented them.

--*John Steinbeck*

Not only our future economic soundness but the very soundness of our democratic institutions depends on the determination of our government to give employment to idle men.

--*Franklin D. Roosevelt*

The best and most beautiful things in the world cannot be seen or even touched - they must be felt with the heart.

--Hellen Keller

We should keep steadily before our minds the fact that Americanism is a question of principle, of purpose, of idealism, of character; that it is not a matter of birthplace, or creed, or line of descent.

--Theodore Roosevelt

Capital punishment is as fundamentally wrong as a cure for crime as charity is wrong as a cure for poverty.

--Henry Ford

Darkness cannot drive out darkness; only light can do that. Hate cannot drive out hate; only love can do that.

--*Martin Luther King, Jr.*

Every reform was once a private opinion.

--*Ralph Waldo Emerson*

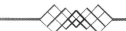

From even the greatest of horrors irony is seldom absent.

--H. P. Lovecraft

I am only an average man but, by George, I work harder at it than the average man.

--*Theodore Roosevelt*

Inflation is as violent as a mugger, as frightening as an armed robber and as deadly as a hit man.

--Ronald Reagan

Magic and all that is ascribed to it is a deep presentiment of the powers of science.

--Ralph Waldo Emerson

Never tell people how to do things. Tell them what to do and they will surprise you with their ingenuity.

--*George S. Patton*

The liberties of a people never were, nor ever will be, secure, when the transactions of their rulers may be concealed from them.

--*James Garfield*

We must accept finite disappointment, but never lose infinite hope.

--Martin Luther King, Jr.

Carry the battle to them. Don't let them bring it to you. Put them on the defensive and don't ever apologize for anything.

--Harry S Truman

Don't be afraid to give up the good to go for the great.

--John D. Rockefeller

For my own part, when I am employed in serving others, I do not look upon myself as conferring favours, but as paying debts. In my travels, and since my settlement, I have received much kindness from men, to whom I shall never have any opportunity of making the least direct return.

--*Benjamin Franklin*

I have been studying the traits and dispositions of the "lower animals" (so called) and contrasting them with the traits and dispositions of man. I find the result humiliating to me.

--*Mark Twain*

Ignorance and bigotry, like other insanities, are incapable of self-government.

--*Thomas Jefferson*

Lost time is never found again.

--Benjamin Franklin

Silence about a thing just magnifies it.

--*Tennessee Williams*

The most difficult place in the world to get a clear and open perspective of the country as a whole is Washington.

--Franklin D. Roosevelt

We must adjust to changing times and still hold to unchanging principles.

--*Jimmy Carter*

Certain events such as love, or a national calamity, or May, bring pressure to bear on the individual, and if the pressure is strong enough, something in the form of verse is bound to be squeezed out.

--John Steinbeck

Everything that we see is a shadow cast by that which we do not see.

--Martin Luther King, Jr.

Having always observed that public works are much less advantageously managed than the same are by private hands, I have thought it better for the public to go to market for whatever it wants which is to be found there; for there competition brings it down to the minimum value.

--*Thomas Jefferson*

I have found the best way to give advice to your children is to find out what they want and then advise them to do it.

--Harry S Truman

If the freedom of speech is taken away then dumb and silent we may be led, like sheep to the slaughter.

--George Washington

It is true that we are weak and sick and ugly and quarrelsome but if that is all we ever were, we would millenniums ago have disappeared from the face of the earth.

--*John Steinbeck*

Nothing is more simple than greatness; indeed, to be simple is to be great.

--Ralph Waldo Emerson

Search others for their virtues, thy self for thy vices.

--Benjamin Franklin

The human mind is a channel through which things-to-be are coming into the realm of things-that-are.

--Henry Ford

Though the will of the majority is in all cases to prevail, that will, to be rightful, must be reasonable.

--*Thomas Jefferson*

We have usurped many of the powers we once ascribed to God... Having taken Godlike power, we must seek in ourselves for the responsibility and the wisdom we once prayed some deity might have.

--John Steinbeck

Charity is injurious unless it helps the recipient to become independent of it.

--John D. Rockefeller

Failure is simply the opportunity to begin again, this time more intelligently.

--Henry Ford

I am a part of everything that I have read.

--Theodore Roosevelt

If ye love wealth greater than liberty, the tranquility of servitude greater than the animating contest for freedom, go ... from us in peace.

--Samuel Adams

Limited minds can recognize limitations only in others.

--Jack London

My favorite things in life don't cost any money. It's really clear that the most precious resource we all have is time.

--*Steve Jobs*

Our Constitution was made only for a moral and religious people. It is wholly inadequate to the government of any other.

--John Adams

People who are most afraid of their dreams convince themselves they don't dream at all.

--John Steinbeck

Religion struck me so vague a thing at best, that I could perceive no advantage of any one system over any other.

--*H. P. Lovecraft*

The first panacea for a mismanaged nation is inflation of the currency; the second is war. Both bring a temporary prosperity; both bring a permanent ruin. But both are the refuge of political and economic opportunists.

--Ernest Hemingway

There never was a good war, or a bad peace.

--*Benjamin Franklin*

Walking with a friend in the dark is better than walking alone in the light.

--Hellen Keller

Is it so bad, then, to be misunderstood? Pythagoras was misunderstood, and Socrates, and Jesus, and Luther, and Copernicus, and Galileo, and Newton, and every pure and wise spirit that ever took flesh. To be great is to be misunderstood.

--*Ralph Waldo Emerson*

Clothes make the man. Naked people have little or no influence in society.

--Mark Twain

Do not think you are going to conceal thoughts by concealing evidence that they ever existed.

--Dwight D. Eisenhower

Greed is merely a species of nearsightedness.

--Henry Ford

I have come to believe that a great teacher is a great artist and that there are as few as there are any other great artists. It might even be the greatest of the arts since the medium is the human mind and spirit.

--*John Steinbeck*

If the American people ever allow private banks to control the issue of currency, first by inflation, then by deflation, the banks and corporations that will grow up around them will deprive the people of all property until their children wake up homeless on the continent their fathers conquered.

--Thomas Jefferson

It must be remembered that there is no real reason to expect anything in particular from mankind; good and evil are local expedients-- or their lack-- and not in any sense cosmic truths or laws.

--H. P. Lovecraft

Many a small thing has been made large by the right kind of advertising.

--Mark Twain

People do not like to think. If one thinks, one must reach conclusions. Conclusions are not always pleasant.

--Hellen Keller

Quality means doing it right when no one is looking.

--Henry Ford

The battle, Sir, is not to the strong alone; it is to the vigilant, the active, the brave.

--*Patrick Henry*

The less there is to justify a traditional custom, the harder it is to get rid of it.

--Mark Twain

Want is a growing giant whom the coat of have was never large enough to cover.

--*Ralph Waldo Emerson*

Death is always and under all circumstances a tragedy, for if it is not, then it means that life itself has become one.

--*Theodore Roosevelt*

He who does something at the head of one regiment, will eclipse him who does nothing at the head of a hundred.

--Abraham Lincoln

I have lived, Sir, a long time, and the longer I live, the more convincing proofs I see of this truth–that God Governs the affairs of men. And if a sparrow cannot fall to the ground without His notice, is it probable that an empire can rise without His aid?

--Benjamin Franklin

It is common sense to take a method and try it: If it fails, admit it frankly and try another. But above all, try something.

--Franklin D. Roosevelt

No new horror can be more terrible than the daily torture of the commonplace.

--H. P. Lovecraft

Only those are fit to live who are not afraid to die.

--Douglas MacArthur

Sometimes a man wants to be stupid if it lets him do a thing his cleverness forbids.

--John Steinbeck

The only things one can admire at length are those one admires without knowing why.

--Eleanor Roosevelt

The sanity of society is a balance of a thousand insanities.

--Ralph Waldo Emerson

Things don't have to change the world to be important.

--Steve Jobs

Wars do not end wars...

--Henry Ford

Courage is resistance to fear, mastery of fear -- not absence of fear.

--*Mark Twain*

Enduring peace cannot be bought at the cost of other people's freedom.

--Franklin D. Roosevelt

Freedom is not a gift bestowed upon us by other men, but a right that belongs to us by the laws of God and nature.

--Benjamin Franklin

Government is merely a servant – merely a temporary servant; it cannot be its prerogative to determine what is right and what is wrong, and decide who is a patriot and who isn't. Its function is to obey orders, not originate them.

--*Mark Twain*

I hope in these days we have heard the last of conformity and consistency. Let the words be gazetted and ridiculous henceforward.

--*Ralph Waldo Emerson*

In the final choice a soldier's pack is not so heavy as a prisoner's chains.

--Dwight D. Eisenhower

Love is the only force capable of transforming an enemy into friend.

--*Martin Luther King, Jr.*

Never miss a good chance to shut up.

--Will Rogers

Ruin looks us in the face if we judge a man by his position instead of judging him by his conduct in that position.

--Theodore Roosevelt

The holy passion of friendship is so sweet and steady and loyal and enduring in nature that it will last through a whole lifetime, if not asked to lend money.

--*Mark Twain*

Too many men are afraid of being fools.

--Henry Ford

We have no government armed with power capable of contending with human passions unbridled by morality and religion.

--John Adams

Discourage litigation. Persuade your neighbors to compromise whenever you can. Point out to them how the nominal winner is often a real loser -- in fees, expenses, and waste of time.

--Abraham Lincoln

Far and away the best prize that life offers is the chance to work hard at work worth doing.

--Theodore Roosevelt

Good breeding consists in concealing how much we think of ourselves and how little we think of the other person.

--*Mark Twain*

Heroes may not be braver than anyone else. They're just braver five minutes longer.

--*Ronald Reagan*

I love to dream, but I never try to dream and think at the same time.

--*H. P. Lovecraft*

In periods where there is no leadership, society stands still.

--*Harry S Truman*

Life isn't hard to manage when you've nothing to lose.

--Ernest Hemingway

Man will ultimately be governed by God or by tyrants.

--Benjamin Franklin

No truth is more evident to my mind than that the Christian religion must be the basis of any government intended to secure the rights and privileges of a free people.

--*Noah Webster*

Plans are nothing; planning is everything.

--Dwight D. Eisenhower

The decline of the Western world began with the invention of the wheel.

--Tennessee Williams

'Tis the good reader that makes the good book.

--Ralph Waldo Emerson

Unexpected money is a delight. The same sum is a bitterness when you expected more.

--Mark Twain

We have no choice, we people of the United States, as to whether or not we shall play a great part in the world. That has been determined to us by fate, by the march of events. We have to play that part. All that we can decide is whether we shall play it well or ill.

--Theodore Roosevelt

Dispositions of the mind, like limbs of the body, acquire strength by exercise.

--Thomas Jefferson

Freedom from effort in the present merely means that there has been effort stored up in the past.

--Theodore Roosevelt

I think that hate is a thing, a feeling, that can only exist where there is no understanding.

--*Tennessee Williams*

Life is not always a matter of holding good cards, but sometimes, playing a poor hand well.

--*Jack London*

Nine-tenths of wisdom is being wise in time.

--Theodore Roosevelt

Pessimism becomes a self-fulfilling prophecy; it reproduces itself by crippling our willingness to act.

--*Howard Zinn*

The Golden Age never was the present age.

--Benjamin Franklin

Today is only one day in all the days that will ever be. But what will happen in all the other days that ever come can depend on what you do today.

--Ernest Hemingway

We could never learn to be brave and patient, if there were only joy in the world.

--*Hellen Keller*

Doing an injury puts you below your enemy; revenging one makes you but even with him; forgiving it sets you above him.

--Benjamin Franklin

Great minds discuss ideas; average minds discuss events; small minds discuss people.

--*Eleanor Roosevelt*

I believe there are more instances of the abridgment of the freedom of the people by the gradual and silent encroachment of those in power, than by violent and sudden usurpation.

--Abraham Lincoln

If I wanted to destroy a nation, I would give it too much and I would have it on its knees, miserable, greedy and sick.

--John Steinbeck

It's a very important thing to learn to talk to people you disagree with.

--Pete Seeger

Mystery creates wonder and wonder is the basis of man's desire to understand.

--Neil Armstrong

I believe that banking institutions are more dangerous to our liberties than standing armies. Already they have raised up a moneyed aristocracy that has set the government at defiance. The issuing power should be taken from the banks and restored to the people, to whom it properly belongs.

--Thomas Jefferson

In my mind nothing is more abhorrent than a life of ease. None of us has any right to ease. There is no place in civilization for the idler.

--Henry Ford

Nothing is more incumbent on the old, than to know when they should get out of the way, and relinquish to younger successors the honors they can no longer earn, and the duties they can no longer perform.

--Thomas Jefferson

The nation behaves well if it treats the natural resources as assets which it must turn over to the next generation increased, and not impaired, in value.

--*Theodore Roosevelt*

There's nothing funnier than the human animal.

--*Walt Disney*

To waste, to destroy, our natural resources, to skin and exhaust the land instead of using it so as to increase its usefulness, will result in undermining in the days of our children the very prosperity which we ought by right to hand down to them amplified and developed.

--Theodore Roosevelt

We are all apprentices in a craft where no one ever becomes a master.

--Ernest Hemingway

Don't loaf and invite inspiration; light out after it with a club, and if you don't get it you will nonetheless get something that looks remarkably like it.

--*Jack London*

He that cannot obey, cannot command.

--Benjamin Franklin

I hope our wisdom will grow with our power, and teach us, that the less we use our power the greater it will be.

--*Thomas Jefferson*

In every battle there comes a time when both sides consider themselves beaten, then he who continues the attack wins.

--Ulysses S. Grant

It's so much darker when a light goes out than it would have been if it had never shone.

--*John Steinbeck*

Never forget that everything Hitler did in Germany was legal.

--Martin Luther King, Jr.

Optimism is the faith that leads to achievement. Nothing can be done without hope and confidence.

--Hellen Keller

The things of the night cannot be explained in the day, because
they do not then exist.

--Ernest Hemingway

There are no easy answers, but there are simple answers. We must have the courage to do what we know is morally right.

--*Ronald Reagan*

Truth is stranger than fiction, but it is because Fiction is obliged to stick to possibilities; Truth isn't.

--*Mark Twain*

We are all civilized people, which means that we are all savages at heart but observing a few amenities of civilized behavior.

--*Tennessee Williams*

Every man is better for a period of work under the open sky.

--Henry Ford

Heaven for climate, Hell for society.

--Mark Twain

I think that people want peace so much that one of these days government had better get out of their way and let them have it.

--*Dwight D. Eisenhower*

If your only goal is to become rich, you will never achieve it.

--John D. Rockefeller

It were not best that we should all think alike; it is difference
of opinion that makes horse races.

--Mark Twain

Nobody will ever deprive the American people of the right to vote except the American people themselves -- and the only way they could do this is by not voting.

--Franklin D. Roosevelt

Pay every debt as if God wrote the bill.

--Ralph Waldo Emerson

Remembering that you are going to die is the best way I know to avoid the trap of thinking you have something to lose. You are already naked. There is no reason not to follow your heart.

--Steve Jobs

The means of defense against foreign danger historically have
become the instruments of tyranny at home.

--James Madison

There are a number of things wrong with Washington. One of them is that everyone is too far from home.

--Dwight D. Eisenhower

We are all of us stars, and we deserve to twinkle.

--Marilyn Monroe

Farming looks mighty easy when your plow is a pencil and you're a thousand miles from the corn field.

--Dwight D. Eisenhower

History, in general, only informs us what bad government is.

--Patrick Henry

I think there is only one quality worse than hardness of heart and that is softness of head.

--Theodore Roosevelt

Income tax has made more liars out of the American people than golf.

--*Will Rogers*

Make your own Bible. Select and collect all the words and sentences that in all your readings have been to you like the blast of a trumpet.

--*Ralph Waldo Emerson*

Nothing really known can continue to be acutely fascinating.

--H. P. Lovecraft

Pilots take no special joy in walking. Pilots like flying.

--Neil Armstrong

Terrorism has replaced Communism as the rationale for the militarization of the country [America], for military adventures abroad, and for the suppression of civil liberties at home. It serves the same purpose, serving to create hysteria.

--Howard Zinn

If a free society cannot help the many who are poor, it cannot save the few who are rich.

--John F. Kennedy

It is unfortunate that the efforts of mankind to recover the freedom of which they have been so long deprived will be accompanied with violence, with errors, and even with crimes. But while we weep over the means, we must pray for the end.

--*Thomas Jefferson*

The unforgivable crime is soft hitting. Do not hit at all if it can be avoided; but never hit softly.

--Theodore Roosevelt

Time is the longest distance between two places.

--Tennessee Williams

We are always getting ready to live, but never living.

--Ralph Waldo Emerson

Human action can be modified to some extent, but human nature cannot be changed.

--Abraham Lincoln

If a nation expects to be ignorant and free, in a state of civilization, it expects what never was and never will be.

--*Thomas Jefferson*

It is only through labor and painful effort, by grim energy and resolute courage, that we move on to better things.

--Theodore Roosevelt

No one who is young is ever going to be old.

--John Steinbeck

The function of education is to teach one to think intensively and to think critically. Intelligence plus character - that is the goal of true education.

--*Martin Luther King, Jr.*

Those who make peaceful revolution impossible will make violent revolution inevitable.

--John F. Kennedy

Unless both sides win, no agreement can be permanent.

--Jimmy Carter

About the Author

John Kerecz has multiple degrees in many different subjects. He has studied martial arts since the age of seven. Now, in his mid-fifties, he enjoys traveling more and finding new adventures. He has flown to space, traveled across the country by motorcycle, and gone shark diving. No moment in life is to be wasted!

Printed in the United States
By Bookmasters